ALSO BY ELIE WIESEL

Hostage

The Sonderberg Case

A Mad Desire to Dance

The Judges

Night

Dawn

The Accident

The Town Beyond the Wall

The Gates of the Forest

The Jews of Silence

Legends of Our Time

A Beggar in Jerusalem

One Generation After

Souls on Fire

The Oath

Ani Maamin (cantata)

Zalmen, or The Madness of God (play)

Messengers of God

A Jew Today

Four Hasidic Masters

The Trial of God (play)

The Testament

Five Biblical Portraits

Somewhere a Master

The Golem (illustrated by Mark Podwal)

The Fifth Son

Against Silence (edited by Irving Abrahamson)

Twilight

The Six Days of Destruction
(with Albert Friedlander)

A Journey of Faith (conversations with
John Cardinal O'Connor)

From the Kingdom of Memory

Sages and Dreamers

The Forgotten

A Passover Haggadah (illustrated by Mark Podwal)

All Rivers Run to the Sea

Memoir in Two Voices (with François Mitterrand)

King Solomon and His Magic Ring
(illustrated by Mark Podwal)

And the Sea Is Never Full

Conversations with Elie Wiesel
(with Richard D. Heffner)

Open Heart

Open Heart

Elie Wiesel

Translated by Marion Wiesel

SCHOCKEN BOOKS | NEW YORK

All rights reserved. Published in the United States by Schocken
Books, a division of Penguin Random House LLC, New York,
and distributed in Canada by Random House of Canada, a
division of Penguin Random House Ltd., Toronto. Originally
published in France as *Coeur ouvert* by Flammarion, Paris, in
2011. Copyright © 2011 by Elirion Associates, Inc. Copyright
© 2011 by Flammarion, Paris. This translation originally
published in hardcover in the United States by Alfred A. Knopf,
a division of Penguin Random House LLC, New York, in 2012.

Schocken Books and colophon are registered trademarks of
Penguin Random House LLC.

The Library of Congress has cataloged the hardcover
Knopf edition as follows:
Wiesel, Elie, [date]
[Coeur ouvert. English]
Open heart / Elie Wiesel ; translated by Marion Wiesel.
p. cm.
1. Wiesel, Elie, [date]. 2. Authors, French—20th century—
Biography. 3. Authors, French—21st century—Biography.
4. Jewish authors—Biography. I. Title.
PQ2683.i32z4612 2012 848'.91403—dc23 [B] 2012038244
Schocken paperback ISBN: 978-0-8052-1258-7
eBook ISBN: 978-0-307-96185-3

Cover photograph by Paul Zimmerman /
WireImage / Getty Images
Cover design by Thomas Colligan

www.schocken.com

Printed in the United States of America
First Schocken Paperback Edition 2015
2 4 6 8 9 7 5 3 1

For Marion and our son, Elisha:

their presence, their love,

helped me overcome the greatest pain

and darkest anguish.

Open Heart

1

J UNE 16, 2011.
      "It's your heart," says the gastroenter-
ologist after performing an endoscopy on me.
   I am surprised: "Not my stomach?"
   For some time now, acid reflux has been
one of my nightmares. My longtime general
practitioner also feels it has contributed to the
various health problems that have afflicted
me for the past several years.
   My wife, Marion, and I have just returned
from Jerusalem, where, every year, we spend
the holiday of Shavuot with close friends. In
keeping with the tradition to which I have
remained faithful, friends and I spent the
night in a yeshiva in the Old City studying
biblical and Talmudic laws and commentaries
dating from the Middle Ages.
   This time, in Jerusalem, it had all gone
well. No terrorist attacks. No border inci-

dents. Even my cursed migraines seemed to respect the sanctity of this night, of this city unlike any other. But now, back in New York, suddenly my body revolts. The new piercing pain in my shoulders rises all the way to my jaw. I swallow a double dose of Nexium, the medicine I take for acid reflux. This time without success.

"No, neither the stomach nor the esophagus," replies the doctor after a moment of silence. "It's certainly the heart." Ominous words, inducing fear and the promise of more pain. Or worse.

2

AS SOON as he receives his colleague's message, my primary care doctor, a cardiologist, reaches me at home. On the phone, he appears to be out of breath; he speaks in a tense, emphatic voice, louder than usual. I have the feeling that he is trying to contain or even hide his nervousness, his concern. Clearly, he is unhappy to have to give me this bad news that will change so many things for me . . .

"I expected a different result," he explains. "But now the situation requires some further tests immediately."

"Yes?"

"Please come to Lenox Hill Hospital right away. I am already there."

I protest: "Why? Because it's the heart? Is it really that urgent? I have never had a problem with my heart. With my head, yes; my stomach too. And sometimes with my eyes. But the heart has left me in peace."

At that, he explodes: "This conversation makes no sense. I am your cardiologist, for heaven's sake! Please don't argue with me! You must take a number of tests that can only be administered at the hospital. Come as quickly as you can! And go to the emergency entrance!"

On occasion, I can be incredibly stupid and stubborn. And so I nevertheless steal two hours to go to my office. I have things to attend to. Appointments to cancel. Letters to sign. People to see—among others, a delegation of Iranian dissidents.

Strange, all this time I am not really worried, though by nature I am rather anxious and pessimistic. My heart does not beat faster. My breathing is normal. No pain. No premonitions. No warning. After all, hadn't I just three days ago gone through a complete checkup with all kinds of tests, including a cardiogram, administered by my physician, the same one who is now ordering me to the hospital? There had been no indication of a coronary problem: no chest pain or feeling of oppression. What has changed so abruptly in my body to destabilize it to this extent?

All right, I'll go to the hospital, since both doctors insist. I don't take anything along. No books, no spare shirt, no toothbrush. Marion says she wants to accompany me. I try to discourage her. In vain.

3

A TEAM of specialists is waiting for me in the emergency room. The very first blood test instantly reveals the gravity of my condition. There is a definite risk of heart attack. The doctors exchange incomprehensible comments in their own jargon. Their conclusion is quick, unambiguous and unanimous: An immediate procedure is required. There can be no delay.

Marion whispers in my ear that we are fortunate; she has just learned that the surgeon who will perform the angiogram is the one who operated on her two years earlier. I remember him, a handsome, strikingly intelligent man. I had been struck by his kindness as much as by his competence.

"I hope," he tells me, "that we will be able to do for you what we succeeded in doing for your wife: to restore a normal flow of blood in the arteries by inserting a stent." But then he adds, looking grave, "I must warn you that we may have to intervene in a more radical way. We will know very soon."

I am drowsy and fight against sleep by trying to follow the brief professional exchanges in the operating room. Actually, I don't understand a word. About an hour later, I hear the surgeon saying, "I am so sorry, I don't have good news for you: Your condition is such that the insertion of a stent won't suffice. You have five blocked arteries. You require open-heart surgery."

I am shaken. Sure, I know that these days open-heart surgery is regularly performed the world over. Dr. Christiaan Barnard's face appears before me; I had met the famous surgeon at a conference in Haifa and we had engaged in a long dialogue on medical ethics, comparing Judaic and Christian points of view. I had looked at his hands, wondering how many human beings owed them their survival.

But now the words "open-heart surgery" are meant for *me*. And they fill me with dread.

"You're lucky. A colleague of mine, an expert in this type of surgery, is at the hospital right now. I have spoken to him. He is ready to operate on you."

"Doctor," I ask, "have you told my wife?"

"No, but I will do it right now."

In a moment he is back: "I've seen Marion. As well as your son, Elisha."

The fact that my beloved son is already at the hospital does not surprise me. Since his earliest childhood, he has always made me proud, always been there for me.

"What do they think?"

"They agree; we have no choice. But the decision is yours alone."

"May I see them?"

Marion and Elisha are not good at hiding their anxiety. Their smiles seem forced. And how am I to hug them without falling apart? Marion, holding back her tears, tries to reassure me: "The doctors are optimistic. The surgeon they propose is world-renowned."

"It will go well," says Elisha. "I know it, Dad. I am convinced of it."

I remain silent.

"Shall we go?" urges the attending physician.

The nurses are ready to push the gurney toward the OR. I steal another glance at the woman with whom I have shared my life for more than forty-two years. So many events, so many discoveries and projects, unite us. All we have done in life we have accomplished together. And now, one more experience.

As the door opens, I look one last time at our son, the fine young man who has justified— and continues to justify—my life and who endows it with meaning and a hereafter.

Through the tears that darken the future, a thought awakens a deeper concern, a deeper sorrow: Shall I see them again?

4

MARION IS here.*

My eyes are closed, but I feel her presence.

I can almost see her.

I think of the extraordinary qualities of this woman. Her strength of character. Her sensitivity. Her intelligence.

I open my eyes.

Marion and Elisha stand next to the gurney, waiting to accompany me to the door of the operating room. Marion looks sad and forlorn. For once there's nothing she can do.

This is the first time I have seen her like this.

She usually knows how to resolve difficult situations. But now she is vainly trying to find words to alleviate my fears. There probably are none.

Any moment now, the door of the OR will

---

*This chapter was translated by the author.

close behind me. Marion is still here, and in a flash I relive our life together, the exceptional moments that have marked it.

I recall our first meeting, at the home of French friends. Love at first sight. Perhaps. Surely on my part. I thought her not only beautiful but superbly intelligent. Hearing her discuss with great passion some Broadway play, I became convinced that I could listen to her for years and years—all my life—without ever interrupting her. I invited her to lunch at an Italian restaurant across from the United Nations. Neither of us touched the food.

Her background? Vienna, then fleeing from place to place; being imprisoned in various camps, including the infamous Camp de Gurs; eventually finding freedom in neutral Switzerland. Finally New York. Everywhere, miracles of adaptation, survival and extraordinary encounters. For years now I have been advising her—begging her, in fact—to write her memoirs. In vain.

We were married in Jerusalem by the late Saul Lieberman, in the Old City (then recently liberated), in the heart of an ancient synagogue, the Ramban, for the most part destroyed by the Jordanian army.

Since then, I cannot imagine my life, my lives, without her.

I owe to her the best translations of my work. Our Foundation for Humanity is fully her responsibility. Since its creation she has given it her energy, talent and imagination.

One day some twenty years ago, Marion called me from Tel Aviv to tell me that she had just visited an "absorption center" for newly arrived Jewish Ethiopian immigrants. She said she would like our foundation to help their children.

Since then, we have opened two large enrichment centers for these children. Marion named the centers Beit Tzipora (House of Tzipora), after my eight-year-old sister who did not return from Auschwitz. When I learned about the name, I remember remaining silent, unable to control my tears.

There are now close to one thousand young people in these centers, and thanks to the help they receive from dedicated teachers, they pass the exams required for entrance to university, essential for a career in Israel.

. . .

All that I have undertaken in my life has been with her. Journeys, projects, dreams of yet more projects—we do it all together. But this time, that is not possible.

Marion attempts a smile. I know that she shares my doubts and fears. The door closes, and I am alone.

5

"IN A few moments, we'll be ready," announces a voice.

Eyes closed, I listen to my heart beating. How much longer? Has the rhythm of the beats slowed down? What about the palpitations?

My thoughts jump wildly; I am disoriented. Where am I? Ideas and images follow one another and collide in my burning head in a frenzied dance. In front of me, the cemetery; behind me, the garden of my childhood. The future is shrinking; the past is dying. And it all unfolds in a dark void. So, I tell myself, I was always told that the void is truly empty, with nothing inside: no flames, no ashes, no wind, no river, no breath and no pain. All nonsense.

I had not even hoped for it—but suddenly I sense the presence of the dead. Have they come to take me with them? Or just to accompany me? Or, why not, to protect me?

And yet, long ago, I did not protect them. I relive the last moments of our shared existence on the train. And then on the infamous ramp built expressly for the new Hungarian transports. I see my little sister, Tsipuka, so beautiful, so innocent. I see her from afar, clutching my mother's hand. I was not with them, at the end.

I see my father at the camp. We were inseparable there. Never had we been so close, so united. Can one die more than once? One could, there. During the death march, the night of the evacuation from Buna. And then during the nocturnal journey in the snow. There again we were together. I protected him and he protected me. Our only disagreement? He wanted me to accept a portion of his miserable bread ration, pretending that he was not hungry. I used the same ploy. Each of us wishing to offer the other one more moment of survival.

And now I shall meet him again; I shall finally die. Absurd, is it not? Long ago, over there, death lay in wait for us at every moment, but it is now, eternities later, that it shall have its way. I feel it.

6

A VOICE penetrates my consciousness: "We are ready."

So am I.

"Would you please count to ten?"

I panic: They are going to put me to sleep—and I shall never wake up again.

"Not yet. Give me another minute. Please. Just a minute."

The silence around us is unreal.

"Why?"

They must be surprised. I don't answer. Shall I explain to them that a practicing Jew, before giving up his soul, if he lacks the time to properly prepare himself, must at least recite a short prayer—a kind of act of faith—a prayer he has known since childhood? Too complicated. To tell them that countless dying victims, martyrs, repeated this prayer before closing their eyes forever: I cannot tell them that.

But I recite it to myself.

Shema Yisrael, hear o Israel, *Adoshem Elokeinu,* God is our God, *Adoshem e'had,* God is one and unique.

"Now I am yours," I say weakly.

"Count. To ten."

I think I stopped before I reached ten.

7

IN THE operating room, I am floating in semi-darkness. Hasty movements, muffled sounds, low voices: all sorts of whispered admonitions as well as encouragement.

All of a sudden, I am afraid. A name has come to my mind, a face: Aviva, a friend of Marion's and the wife of our friend Émil Najar, former Israeli ambassador to Rome and Tokyo. She too had suffered heart problems, and she too underwent surgery. But she did not get up from the table.

To chase this onset of anxiety, I let my thoughts take me back to a distant past. I am eight or nine, and a doctor, my cousin Oscar, is removing my tonsils. During the operation I take refuge in heaven, where angels are running back and forth, paying me no heed. Clearly, they do not think me worthy of their attention. I recall this dream because when I awoke, I told it to Oscar.

A more serious operation: I am ten or eleven years old, and I am on a train with my parents. It is Shabbat, a day on which, in principle, a practicing Jew may not travel. However, our close neighbor, the Rabbi of Borshe, a brother of the famed Rabbi Israël of Wizsnitz, had granted my parents permission to violate the sanctity of the Seventh Day to take me to Satmar. My appendix has to be removed, and the only Jewish hospital is located there. The surgery takes place the next day. They try to put me to sleep with ether, but I refuse to inhale. Amazingly, what I remember most vividly after all this time—decades—is the young and beautiful nurse with long dark hair and a warm smile. She reassures me: "Let me put you to sleep." I let her. She takes care of me the entire following week. If at that time I could have expressed myself better, and had not been afraid of words, I would have admitted to myself that I had fallen in love with her. For a long time, I was ashamed when I met her again and again in my adolescent dreams.

Suddenly, I realize that I am in the hands of the surgeon and must face the truth: When

I fall asleep, it may well be forever. Am I afraid to die? In the past, whenever I thought of death, I was not frightened. Hadn't I lived with death, even *in* death? Why should I be afraid now?

8

YET, THIS is not how I imagined my end. And in no way did I feel ready.

So many things still to be achieved. So many projects to be completed. So many challenges yet to face. So many prayers yet to compose, so many words yet to discover, so many courses yet to give, so many lessons yet to receive.

This is when I learned much about myself and my surroundings. In particular, I learned that, sadly, when the body becomes a prisoner of its pain, a pill or an injection is more helpful than the most brilliant philosophical idea.

There are still so many things I want to share with my two grandchildren, for whom my love is without limits.

When Elijah smiles at me, I know that happiness exists after all.

His little sister, Shira, both charming and

authoritarian, orders me around and makes me laugh.

To watch them play together, to listen to Elijah reading to his sister, is the most beautiful present I could receive.

Am I ready to lose their love?

9

THE PAIN of the incision wakes me up. As well as the surgeon's voice, perceived through heavy fog:

"It's over. Everything is fine. You'll live."

His face! I shall never forget the smile on his face. My surgeon is happy. Yes, happy to have brought back to life a human being he had never met before. He tells me, "You've come back from far away."

A question: Had I really dreamed during the operation? Had my brain really continued to function while my heart had stopped?

I later learned the exact procedure of bypass surgery: dramatic and impressive on every level.

I didn't know, I couldn't know, just how complicated it is, with risks and dangers that defy imagination. For the layman that I am, this surgery is not unlike a walk on the moon. There is the frightening discovery of the need to temporarily stop the heart, to replace it with a machine while the surgeon operates. He begins by opening the thoracic cage—via an incision down the entire length of the sternum—and then makes a second incision on the inside of one leg in order to remove a vein that will replace the blocked arteries.

I was "coming back" from far away, very far away indeed. And I could just as easily have stayed on the other side.

I am overcome with a feeling of gratitude.

Still under the influence of anesthesia, I try to whisper: "Thank you. Thank you, doctor."

At that moment, did I think of thanking God as well? After all, I owe Him that much. But I am not sure that I did. At that precise moment, only the surgeon—His messenger, no doubt—moved me to gratitude.

I ask weakly, so weakly that I'm afraid I'm not heard, "Do they know?"

No need to be more specific; do Marion and Elisha know that I'm all right?

Yes. Even before I woke completely, the

surgeon himself went to give them the good news.

We are reunited an hour later. The three of us, in our own way, try to cover up our emotion.

IS IT dawn or dusk? Elisha is with me, in my room. How long has he been here?

I glance at the clock on the wall. Around me and my son, objects dissolve. "Elisha," I say breathlessly.

I don't know if he hears me. But it does me good to pronounce his name. As always, I cling to him to defeat anxiety, and that helps me pull myself together.

Now too?

As always.

I perceive voices coming from the hallway. But only his has meaning and purpose.

NUMEROUS SCENES appear before me. Elisha as a child, an adolescent, an adult.

Elisha's birth changed my life. From that moment, I felt more concerned and responsible than ever before. This tiny creature looking at me without seeing me would have to be protected. And the best way to protect him would be to change the world in which he would grow up.

For the circumcision ceremony we had invited friends, among them the great violinist Isaac Stern, the philosopher Rabbi Abraham Joshua Heschel, many writers and survivors. All had come, naturally, for legend tells us that this is the only invitation one may not decline, since a circumcision always takes place "in the presence" of the patriarch Abraham and the prophet Elijah.

I remember it as if it were yesterday.

We had also invited a number of Hasidim from Brooklyn, and when the name of the newborn—Shlomo Elisha son of Eliezer, son of Shlomo—was pronounced for the first time, an old Hasid cried out, "A name has come back to us." And he and some of the other Hasidim formed a circle and began to dance around, and in honor of, the newly arrived Jew. I, who do not know how to dance, joined in.

After the ceremony, I sat down and wrote a letter to my friend Georges Levitte, one of the great intellectuals of France, father of Jean-David Levitte, the future diplomatic counsel to Jacques Chirac and then to Nicolas Sarkozy. We were close friends and saw each other often whenever I was in Paris.

Some time earlier, he had heard me on the radio saying that I planned never to marry and surely not to have children. Why? I quoted a Talmudic sage: "When God punishes a sinful world, it is wiser not to marry." Georges did not agree and disapproved of my response. He felt I had no right to discourage young people and thus contribute to their despair.

Our discussion had lasted several hours, and we had parted with neither having convinced the other.

My letter was brief: "You were right. My son bears my father's name, Shlomo. One more name regained, for we have lost too many. He is also called Elisha."

To say that the love I felt for my son was filled with fervor and hope would not be enough. I would spend hours and hours just looking at him. To leave him for more than a day was painful. And whenever I had to go out of town, I somehow managed to return before Shabbat. To hold him in my arms as I made Kiddush fulfilled a strong emotional need.

Mornings, when he left for nursery school, Marion and I would walk him to the yellow school bus. As I watched the vehicle draw away, my heart beat faster. I see him still, his little hand motioning to us. And deep inside me I prayed to God to protect him.

After graduating from college, Elisha decided to go to Israel for a semester, to join other young non-Israelis in a training camp for the Israel Defense Forces. On the way to the airport, I found myself repeating the prayer my mother recited at the end of every Shabbat, imploring God to bless our house and our family.

"ELISHA," I say very quietly.

My son hears me: "What can I do for you?"

During his first year at Yale, Elisha studied philosophy, history and literature. Secretly, I was hoping that he would follow in my footsteps, but he was recruited by Wall Street. The economy, the markets: alien territories to me.

And now he is a father. In my view, the best father in the world.

I motion him to approach. Now he is very close to my bed. He takes my hand in his and caresses it gently. I try to squeeze his hand but don't succeed. I know that he wishes to transmit to me his strength, his faith in my recovery.

BY DINT of searching for him in the past, suddenly I picture him as an orphan. I remember promising myself to watch over him even after my death, and here I am, on the threshold of the beyond.

Have I followed the advice of the Talmudic sage: "It is incumbent on you to live as if you were to die the next day"?

The first question the angel asks the dead is "Were you honest in your dealings with others?" And then: "Did you truly live waiting for the Messiah?"

When will the angel interrogate me?

Images rise up from ancient midrashic and mystical sources, crowding my brain and my memory. In my adolescence at the yeshiva, they used to make me tremble. Many texts describe the beyond. Few take place in paradise; most unfold in hell. The sinners and their punishment in the flames. Their deafening screams, their unimaginable suffering, which ends only with the arrival of Shabbat.

Am I, in fact, already on the other side? If not, would I have been permitted a glimpse into the beyond?

I am lying on my hospital bed, but it is hell. My skin is ripping apart; my entire body is aflame. I see myself in hell, ruled by cruel, pitiless angels. My head filled with medieval descriptions of unimaginable punishments, I think I know—I do know—what takes place in these dreadful abysses.

Tears and screams fill the subterranean hells.

That is the fiery universe inflicted upon sinners. Men hanged by their tongues, women by their breasts. I try to identify them; in vain. Their faces are disfigured, unrecognizable. Is mine among them?

And then my gaze turns to the others, the Just: They are imploring the supreme Judge to show mercy to His people in exile. The ancestors, the prophets, the visionaries and their friends, the masters and the poets—one more step ahead and I shall be their student; I shall be one of them.

Am I ready?

14

IS ONE ever ready?

Some of the ancient Greek philosophers, as well as some Hasidic masters, claimed to have spent their lifetimes preparing for death.

Well, the Jewish tradition, which is my own, counsels another way: We sanctify life, not death. "*Ubakharta bakhaim,*" says Scripture: "You shall choose life" and the living. With the promise to live a better, more moral, more humane life.

That is what man's efforts should be directed to. To save the life of a human being, whomever he or she may be, wherever he or she is from, a Jew has the right to transgress the strictest of the Torah's laws. That is what I learned in heder when I was very young, and later at the yeshiva, and later still by studying the sacred books. Death—any death— renders impure all who come in contact with it. Even the death of Moses, which is why God undertook to bury him Himself.

Of course, we must accept the idea—the reality—that every man is mortal. But Jewish law teaches us that death is not meant to guide us; it is life that will show us the way. And the choice is never ours. All decisions are made up above on Rosh Hashanah, the New Year. On that day—this is what our prayers affirm—God inscribes in the Book of Life all that will happen to us in the year to come: who shall know joy and who shall experience sorrow; who shall become ill and who shall live and who shall die.

Evidently, I have prayed poorly, lacking concentration and fervor; otherwise, why would the Lord, by definition just and merciful, punish me in this way?

Hardly have I formulated this conclusion than I reject it: Were it valid today, how much more valid it would have been then, *there*.

15

SUCH ARE the thoughts that the patient, a prisoner of his condemned body, confronting his fate, is experiencing with ferocious intensity. As I face the gravity of this moment, I feel the need to search my soul.

I am eighty-two years old. As it has often before, and now more so than ever, the fact that I am who I am leads me to look back: What have I done, and what have I toiled to do, during this long journey filled with dreams and challenges?

Strange, I suddenly remember Baudelaire's outcry in his *Mon cœur mis à nu* (My Heart Laid Bare): "There exist in every man, at every hour, two simultaneous impulses; one leading toward God, the other toward Satan." Have I distinguished the path to Good from the one leading to Evil?

My life unfolds before me like a film:

landscapes from my childhood; adventures in faraway, sometimes exotic places; my first masters, followed by my first moments of adolescent religious ecstasy as I and my friends at the yeshiva received from our old masters the keys that open the secret doors of mystical truths.

Have I performed my duty as a survivor? Have I transmitted all I was able to? Too much, perhaps? Were some of the mystics not punished for having penetrated the secret garden of forbidden knowledge?

To begin, I attempted to describe the time of darkness. Birkenau, Auschwitz, Buchenwald. A slight volume: *Night*. First in Yiddish, *"And the world remained silent,"* in which every sentence, every word, reflects an experience that defies all comprehension. Even had every single survivor consecrated a year of his life to testifying, the result would probably still have been unsatisfactory. I rarely reread myself, but when I do, I come away with a bitter taste in my mouth: I feel the words are not right and that I could have said it better. In my writings about the Event, did I commit a sin by saying too much, while fully knowing that no person who did not experience the proximity of death there can ever understand what we, the survivors, were subjected to from morning till night, under a silent sky?

I have written some fifty works—most dealing with topics far removed from the one I continue to consider essential: the victims' memory. I believe that I have done all I could to prevent it from being cheapened or altogether stifled, but was it enough? And if I often published works—articles, novels—on other themes, I did so in order not to remain its prisoner. My battle against the trivialization and banalization of Auschwitz in film and on television resulted in my gaining not a few enemies. To my thinking, it was my duty to show that the sum of all the suffering and deaths is an integral part of the texts we revere.

In my imagination, I turn the pages.

The Bible and the prophets, the Talmud and Hasidism, the Baal Shem Tov and his disciples, mysticism and ethics: All that I received from my masters, present and gone,

I attempted to transmit. Involuntarily, unwittingly, my experience of what some among us so poorly call the Shoah, or Holocaust, slipped in, here and there, between the lines, into the silences that surround a text. Just as I inevitably situate my novels in the shadow of invisible flames. But have I been prudent enough?

My very first works of fiction are set not during the Event, but after. Why?

In *Dawn*—about the clandestine struggle of the Jews against the British army in Palestine—a survivor of the death camps is ordered to execute a British officer.

In *Day,* a young journalist is run over by a taxi in New York. Accident or attempted suicide?

The Town Beyond the Wall? A book on man's fascination with madness.

The Gates of the Forest? An homage to friendship, and the story of a young orphan who pretends to be deaf and mute and who is given the part of Judas in a Passion Play at school.

I often think of these entirely fictional

works, losing myself in an elusive elsewhere, searching for my inner compass.

The Jews of Silence, set in Communist Russia, derives from another source. That work makes me proud, for it helped brave men and women free themselves of dictatorship and join their brothers and sisters in the land of our ancestors.

The same is true of my novel *The Forgotten,* which deals with Alzheimer's disease and the fear of forgetting. I compare the patient to a book whose pages are torn out day after day, one by one, until all that remains is the cover. I wonder whether this disease could strike an entire community. Or an entire era. In Jewish religious texts, there is great emphasis on the fact that the Lord forgets nothing. Is that because the possibility of divine neglect is not excluded from our subconscious? And so it is with our devotion to the Holy City. King David, in his Psalms, sings: "If I forget thee, Jerusalem . . ." I am his distant disciple, and I say it in my own way.

A Beggar in Jerusalem—I shall bring the

title character along when I appear before the celestial Tribunal as a witness for my defense. I had met him in front of the Wall during the Six-Day War. There I stood, hands outstretched, my soul on fire, writing with my lips. I found him handsome, this beggar who sought to explain to me the miraculous aspect of the Jewish army's great victory over its enemies. You see, he said, our army included another six million souls. . . . That evening, alone in my hotel room, I wrote down all I had heard and felt it with renewed fervor.

The Testament represents my attempt to unmask communism—in particular, the liquidation of the great Jewish novelists and poets during the Stalin era. Begun as a messianism without God, invented as a marvelous message of comradeship, a noble concept of brotherly humanism, communism was transformed by Stalin into a gigantic laboratory for deception, torture and murder.

What to say about "Ani Maamin"? "I believe in the coming of the Messiah," declared Maimonides, and we repeat it with him. "Even though he may be late—and he shall be so indefinitely—I shall go on waiting for him every day." It is a song of deep and gracious beauty. It speaks of a secret hope without which life would become but a handful of dust. It is a song I learned at the Rabbi of Wizsnitz's court, to which my mother and I had journeyed to celebrate the Shabbat Shira, the morning service during which we read of the miraculous Red Sea crossing.

On that day, we had met the Rabbi's nephew, who had escaped, no one knew how, from a ghetto in Poland. At that time, Hungarian Jews had no inkling of the tragedy that was about to befall their communities. Auschwitz and Treblinka were unknown names to us.

This nephew, what is he doing in my hospital room? Why do I see him now just as I did long ago at his uncle's? On that day, this small, skinny, melancholic young man, who seemed locked in his solitude, never stopped moving his lips as he prayed in silence. What made me think of that afternoon, between the service of Minha and the Third Mystical Meal, when the students surrounding him asked him to tell us what happened to him? He had refused to answer. We insisted. But he remained huddled in a corner, a shadow among so many shadows, and remained silent. Until, in the end, he shook himself and gave in: "Fine," he said very softly, "I shall tell you." And he began to sing "Ani Maamin," the most beautiful, most moving *nigun* I had ever heard. He added nothing: For him, the song said it all.

Shall I be able to sing up above? Shall I too be able to intone this *nigun* that contains all that I have tried to express in my writings?

16

THE YEAR 2011 will forever remain for me a year of malediction.

In mid-January, Marion and I were in Florida. For several years I have been co-teaching a class in philosophy, history and literature with a local colleague at a small, prestigious college.

Ten days after I arrived in Florida, I became ill. The doctors diagnosed double pneumonia and ordered what we thought would be a week of hospitalization. After I'd been at the hospital for a few days, my condition worsened. I asked Marion to do everything, anything, to convince the doctors to allow me to leave. She argued that she was afraid I would become seriously depressed and begged them to find a way to care for me at our hotel.

At first the doctors would not hear of it.

They said that neither of us had any idea of the gravity of my condition. "Pneumonia, and what's more, double pneumonia, requires constant supervision. The patient requires medications that need to be administered intravenously. Impossible outside the hospital."

In the end, Marion proposed turning our hotel room into a veritable hospital room, complete with round-the-clock nurses. Even I was surprised when the doctors accepted.

But I was growing weaker and weaker. Ridiculously, all I was concerned about was that, for the first time in my professional life, I had to interrupt my courses, and my students were taken over by my colleague. I felt unhappy and guilty, for teaching and writing remain my true passions. When I miss a class, I am probably more disappointed than anyone else.

Only later did I learn that during those days and nights, my life had been in danger. In truth, I had not given it any thought. In spite of the difficulty I had breathing because my lungs were filled with fluid, I was still able to read, reflect, dream.

After a few months back in New York, I resumed my "normal" existence. If someone had suggested to me that the real ordeal still lay ahead, hidden in my chest, I probably would have called him a nasty prophet.

17

YES, I have written much, and yet, at this stage of my life, at the very threshold of the great portal, I feel that I have not even begun. Too late?

Similarly, I question my many other activities. For example, in my combat against hatred, which I wished to be unrelenting, did I in fact invest enough time, enough energy, in denouncing fanaticism in its various guises? Evidently not, since all of us who have fought the battle must now admit defeat.

At the time of the liberation of the camps, I remember, we were convinced that after Auschwitz there would be no more wars, no more racism, no more hatred, no more anti-Semitism. We were wrong. This produced a feeling close to despair. For if Auschwitz could not cure mankind of racism, was there any chance of success ever? The fact is, the world has learned nothing. Otherwise, how is one to comprehend the atrocities committed in Cambodia, Rwanda, Bosnia . . . ?

I have initiated many actions, in countless locations, with many companions. And fought so many battles. Was it all in vain?

What shall I say to God? That I was also counting on His help? Shall I have the nerve to reproach Him for His incomprehensible silence while Satan was winning his victories? While my father, Shlomo son of Eliezer and Nissel, lay dying on his cot?

Suddenly, here is my father; he too is in my room.

I see three images in one: my father in Buchenwald, my father in the present and one image from my visit to the camp two years ago. There are other people around us, mostly unknown except for one: President Barack Obama, who had invited me to accompany him to Buchenwald. Had he been told that there were in fact two camps, known as large and small? In any case, we visited the small one, the more lethal one. When I left New York to meet him and his entourage on their official visit in Germany, I didn't think I would have to make any formal remarks. Marion thought that I would, and I was convinced that, for once, she was wrong, since my name did not appear on the program. She was right. As he was about to begin his speech, the president leaned toward me and whispered, "In this place, it is you who must have the last word." I improvised, speaking about a son's duty to visit his father's grave to meditate. I remember saying that my father has no grave, that his grave is in the largest cemetery in history, the one that is in heaven. That he died not far from here, in this camp, and that I was there too, close to him and yet so far. When he called me, I had neither the strength nor the courage to go to him. It was the first time I had disobeyed him, and I confessed that I was paralyzed by fear.

And now, on my hospital bed, it is my turn to call him.

And of course my father responds.

18

IN TRUTH, my father never leaves me. Nor do my mother and little sister. They have stayed with me, appearing in every one of my tales, in every one of my dreams. In everything I teach.

After surgery, as I lie on my bed fighting off pain, I review what I have accomplished as a teacher. For the past forty years, I have lived among the young, and I fully know that I have received more from them than I have given. If I could teach them one last time, what would I say?

The midrash tells us that there is an academy in heaven. And that God Himself studies there with our masters. Some sources affirm that the Messiah is there, seated at the same table as the masters and their disciples. Will they allow me to join them? I am counting on my grandfather Reb Dodye Feig to intercede for me.

For the moment of joining them has almost arrived; I am convinced of it. I feel it.

Once again I appeal to the memory of my parents and grandparents. Even though none of them ever reached my age, I should like to prolong my life by a few years, by a few months or at least by a few moments.

For there are so many unfinished projects! A study on asceticism, initiated a long time ago because the concept of accepted, invoked suffering has preoccupied me since the end of the war. I also would like to develop the ideas advanced in an already-published book, *Somewhere a Master,* in which we find yesterday's masters and today's side by side: Moses, who remains our master; Rabbi Akiba, our steadfast friend; and so many others, including Maimonides, Rabbi Bahya Ibn Pekudah, the Baal Shem Tov, the Gaon of Vilna, Rav Shushani and Rav Saul Lieberman.

Even in my present state, my head is bursting with so many questions: How does one become a master? How does one simultaneously stimulate and appease the intellectual and spiritual thirst of a young student? Interestingly, in Hasidism, it is the disciple who chooses his master, not the other way around.

And there is so much more I'd like to say on another topic: friendship. I devoted a course to it at Boston University, a course that was most of all a celebration, for friendship contains an element of immortality. A broken friendship results in deep sadness, deeper even than what we may feel at the end of love.

Probably none of those projects will become realized. I have had my doubts for some time because, sadly, my body, which remains an enigma for me, often refuses to cooperate. And has, in fact, already played a number of tricks on me.

For example, as a child, I suffered from severe migraines. As did my parents. They took me from doctor to doctor, in Sighet and as far away as Budapest. But no specialist, no medication, provided relief. The term "genetic" was uttered. And then, oddly, my headaches stopped the night of my arrival in Birkenau. And returned, as intensely as ever, the morning of my arrival in Ecouis, the first of the children's homes that welcomed me in France in 1945.

No professor of medicine, no neurologist, in Paris or in New York, has ever been able to explain this phenomenon to me.

My body decided to be incomprehensible. Like the soul, it remains a mystery.

19

HOSPITAL LIFE is something I am familiar
with.

July 1956. Correspondent for the Israeli
daily *Yedioth Ahronoth* at the United Nations,
I have just arrived from Paris. Every evening
I walk over to the New York Times Building
to buy the first edition of the paper, which—
truth be told—is helpful to all foreign jour-
nalists in their work.

That particular evening, clutching the
newspaper under my arm, I cross Times
Square, heading for the telegraphic bureau
from which I dispatch my daily cable. That
cable is never sent: I am run over by a taxi.
Multiple fractures of the hip, the vertebrae,
the ankles.

The surgery lasts several hours. When I
awaken, a cast is covering my entire body
except my head and arms. For three long

months, a hospital room becomes my headquarters. I need assistance to move or accomplish any task. I am unable to change position without calling for help.

Fortunately, I have made a few friends among my United Nations colleagues and so, from morning till night, I am rarely alone. I especially remember Daniel Morgaine (*France-Soir*) and Alexander Zauber (*Iton Meyuchad*). The latter, endowed with a magnificent sense of humor, loves to make me laugh. And while laughing makes me feel better, it also hurts.

On his first visit, he wants to know everything about my accident. I describe my various fractures, and as I mention each one, he nods and says, "It could be worse." I have terrible headaches: "It could be worse." My left ankle is broken: "It could be worse." My knees are on fire: "It could be worse." Surprised and somewhat annoyed, at one point I cannot hold back: "Really, Alexander, what could be worse?"

And with a serious face, my friend murmurs, "It could have been me."

Another time, I remind him, a former yeshiva student, of a prayer that as a child I recited every morning: "Blessed be Thou, Lord, who has created man wisely. In his body, there are a multitude of arteries, cavities and openings: if but one of them were to be blocked or damaged, he could not survive an hour."

And I add, "Only now do I understand those words."

Alexander's response: "If you don't watch out, you'll discover other similar prayers. And the Lord will help you to better understand other aspects of your body."

Several decades later, I discover things my body has kept secret all my life. Do I really need to know them?

20

ONCE BACK in my room, I give in to fatigue. Everything exhausts me. To breathe, to open my eyes, to think—everything brings renewed agony. Am I out of danger? Not yet. They say so over and over. My wife and my son try to reassure me. Their voices reach me from afar: They are asking me whether I would like them to stay overnight, but a physician's aide advises against it; the powerful medications will make me fall asleep soon. I hear them discuss: They would like to stay at least an hour or two. Their presence does me good. I'd like to intervene in their exchange, but a large tube has just been removed from my throat and it hurts.

In spite of the sedation and tranquilizers, I sleep poorly. Nurses and nurse's aides constantly manipulate my body, turning it in every direction. Multiple injections, unending blood tests, checkups from top to bottom. No sooner do I close my eyes than I must open them again. My lids remain half closed. I think I dreamed, but I can't recall clearly what the dreams were about. I do remember their color, though: gray-black ashes and an incandescent flame rising from a gigantic chimney consuming rows upon rows of books.

Am I really saved? For good? I doubt it. Nothing seems real to me. Still, death has evidently decided not to claim my body as yet. A strange heaviness overwhelms me. It is in my chest, my head, and it pulls me down. Toward the void.

I feel the proximity of the dark, implacable enemy. I no longer know where I am going, where I am, who I am. Nor even what I want. The doctors try to convince me that from now on, for a few days, a few weeks, I must be patient, that the feeling of being cut into pieces will disappear. But when? Tomorrow. The day after tomorrow. If only I could sleep a week, perhaps even a month.

A lingering doubt: What if the doctors are

hiding the truth from me? What if, in fact, I am dying? It could still happen: I may die any minute. But I am not dead yet. What does being resuscitated mean if not rediscovering one's future?

21

THE OPPRESSION lasts thirty-six hours, perhaps two days. An eternity during which I
can do nothing without help. Huge bandages
cover my chest and the inside of my right
leg. Electrocardiograms constantly control
my heart rhythm. Attached to my body are
long cables to analyze and measure the func-
tioning of my vital organs. True, I had been
warned that I would lose all notion of time
and reality, except that every vanished reality
makes way for another. Indefinitely.

On the third day, I am at last able to leave my
bed. Then my room, to walk a few steps in
the hallway. The state of my health improves,
but the discomfort due to the incisions in the
chest and leg persists. Yes, I do have medications, but they upset my stomach. It seems my
brain is affected as well, for I am certainly

thinking less clearly. I feel removed in time and space; I do not recognize myself. Who am I? What have I become? I know that I have escaped death. I also know that my life will never be the same again.

22

AND GOD in all that?

Am I asking myself that terrible question to chase away my anxiety and my pain?

Now that I am confined to the hospital bed, that question arises again, obsesses me as it haunts all I have written. And, lover of insoluble philosophical problems that I am, I remain frustrated.

A great journalist, a friend, in a televised conversation, asked me what I would say to God as I stood before Him I answered with one word: "Why?"

And God's answer? If, in His kindness, as we say, He actually communicated His answer, I don't recall it.

The Talmud tells me: Moses is present as Rabbi Akiba gives a lecture on the Bible. And Moses asks God, "Since this master is so erudite, why did You give the Law to me rather than to him?" And God answers harshly: "Be quiet. For such is my will!" Some time later, Moses is present at Rabbi Akiba's terrible torture and death at the hands of Roman soldiers. And he cries out, "Lord, is this Your reward to one who lived his entire life celebrating Your Law?" And God repeats His answer with the same harshness: "Be quiet. For such is my will!"

What will His answer be now, to make me be quiet?

And where shall I find the audacity and the strength to not accept it?

And yet, once I have left the antechamber of death, I ponder the question again. Why this illness? These pains, why did I deserve them? Even the possible success of the surgery leads me to inquire: "And God in all this?" Merciful God—as we say—did He not, after all, intervene and lend a hand to the surgeon? But again why, for what purpose?

When I was a child, I situated God exclusively in all that is Good. In all that is sacred. In all that makes man worthy of salvation. Could it be that for God, Evil represents just another path leading to Good?

In truth, for the Jew that I am, Auschwitz is not only a human tragedy but also—and most of all—a theological scandal. For me, it is as impossible to accept Auschwitz with God as without God. But then how is one to understand His silence?

As I try to explain God's presence in Evil, I suffer. And search for reasons that would allow me to denounce it. Thoughts I expressed already in *Night,* in particular in the passage that describes a Rosh Hashanah service in Buna:

> Never shall I forget the nocturnal silence that deprived me for all eternity of the desire to live. Never shall I forget those moments that murdered my God and my soul and turned my dreams to ashes. Never shall I forget those things, even were I condemned to live as long as God Himself.

But a few lines later I describe how during the same service I recite the traditional prayers and litanies, and proclaim my faith in Him, God of Abraham, Isaac and Jacob. . . .

I confess to having rebelled against the Lord, but I have never repudiated Him.

Having studied the sublime, enchanting texts of the prophets, I make mine Jeremiah's Lamentations, evoking the destruction of the first Temple of Jerusalem:

"You have killed [Your children] without mercy!"

"You have assassinated [Your people] without compassion!"

What? God, assassin? True, some of us protested against the divine silence. But none of us had the audacity to call God "assassin"!

On the third day, I feel the need to say my daily prayers. I ask Marion to bring me my tallith and tefillin.

To thank Him? To explain to God that I believe in Him in spite of Himself? My thoughts are still too nebulous to formulate a valid response on the subject of the Almighty.

I do, however, find a response, more personal perhaps: namely, that my commitment is an affirmation of my fidelity to the religious practice of my parents and theirs. If I observe the laws of the Torah by putting on the tefillin, it is because my father and grandfather, and theirs, did so. I refuse to be the last in a line going back very far in my memory and that of my people.

I know this answer is in no way satisfactory, or perhaps not even valid. But it is the only one.

All my life, until today, I have been content to ask questions. All the while knowing that the real questions, those that concern the Creator and His creation, have no answers. I'll go even farther and say that there is a level at which only the questions are eternal; the answers never are.

And so, the patient that I am, more charitable, repeats, "Since God is, He is to be found in the questions as well as in the answers."

ONE DAY at the beginning of my convales-
cence, little Elijah, five years old, comes to
pay me a visit. I hug him and tell him, "Every
time I see you, my life becomes a gift."

He observes me closely as I speak and then,
with a serious mien, responds:

"Grandpa, you know that I love you, and
I see you are in pain. Tell me: If I loved you
more, would you be in less pain?"

I am convinced God at that moment is
smiling as He contemplates His creation.

24

PHYSICIANS WARNED me that the feelings of weakness and fatigue would last long after I left the hospital. And so, for several weeks I walk like an old man—after all, I am only eighty-two! I have to make a considerable effort to hold myself straight. Every few steps, I have to stop, short of breath, and rest a moment until I am able to go on. Also, the pain in my chest continues to prevent me from sleeping.

Among the interdictions imposed by the physician: no smoking. But I have not smoked for forty-two years, since I married. No alcohol either. It happens that I don't drink; I never did. No exercise. Never did that either.

And then came the warning: "A bypass brings with it deep depression." Why? I don't know; it probably is linked to the many mysteries of the heart. In my case, it didn't happen.

As yet.

A CREDO that defines my path:

I belong to a generation that has often felt abandoned by God and betrayed by mankind. And yet, I believe that we must not give up on either.

Was it yesterday—or long ago—that we learned how human beings have been able to attain perfection in cruelty? That for the killers, the torturers, it is normal, thus human, to act inhumanely? Should one therefore turn away from humanity?

The answer, of course, is up to each of us. We must choose between the violence of adults and the smiles of children, between the ugliness of hate and the will to oppose it. Between inflicting suffering and humiliation on our fellow man and offering him the solidarity and hope he deserves. Or not.

I know—I speak from experience—that even in darkness it is possible to create light and encourage compassion. That it is possible to feel free inside a prison. That even in exile, friendship exists and can become an anchor. That one instant before dying, man is still immortal.

There it is: I still believe in man in spite of man. I believe in language even though it has been wounded, deformed and perverted by the enemies of mankind. And I continue to cling to words because it is up to us to transform them into instruments of comprehension rather than contempt. It is up to us to choose whether we wish to use them to curse or to heal, to wound or to console.

As a Jew, I believe in the coming of the Messiah. But of course this does not mean that the world will become Jewish; just that it will become more welcoming, more human. I belong, after all, to a generation that has learned that whatever the question, indifference and resignation are not the answer.

Illness may diminish me, but it will not destroy me. The body is not eternal, but the idea of the soul is. The brain will be buried, but memory will survive it.

Such is the miracle: A tale about despair becomes a tale against despair.

26

THIS OPEN-HEART introspection would not be complete if I did not ask a last question: Have I changed? With what my heart has gone through, during and since the hospitalization of June 16, 2011, after the forays into the unknown and the explorations of the depths of my being, am I still the same? The pain and its memory, the nightmares real and imagined, the necessary and inevitable medications must have affected my brain and—why not?—my soul.

Is it possible to come so close to the end without something essential changing inside us? Has my perception of death, and thus of life, not changed? Are there deeds that someone who has undergone this experience would no longer commit, or, at the least, would accomplish differently?

I believe that the answer is yes.

This is true even from a practical point of view. I have learned that I must refuse certain foods, avoid certain movements, accept certain situations without getting upset.

And yet I have essentially remained the same. It might seem that I am not the man I was before June 16, 2011, but on a level close to the absolutes that are life and death, I have remained the same. What is different is that I now know that every moment is a new beginning, every handshake a promise.

I know that every quest implicates the *other,* just as every word can become prayer. If life is not a celebration, why remember it? If life—mine or that of my fellow man—is not an offering to the *other,* what are we doing on this earth?

For I have learned, over the course of years, to observe man's mystical capacities, and, in spite of the contradictions inherent to my testimonies, I persist in believing in them.

For my conscience—thus, my being—continues to carry the past into the present. If what I experienced long ago in the distant landscape of the disappeared has not changed me, why would this new ordeal succeed?

I know that eternities ago, the day after the liberation, when some of us had to choose between anger and gratitude, my choice was the right one.

Postscript

ONE YEAR later.

I try to go back to my so-called normal life. Not easy. Physically, the doctors' predictions seem correct: My fatigue is clinging to me, unrelenting in its pursuit of me, even into my sleep. It is as difficult to overcome as it is to get used to. Strange, I even dream slowly, and the events that dominate the news seem to move reluctantly into my thoughts.

I walk ten minutes from my apartment to my office and I am out of breath. There is even a difference in my reading: Turning the pages is no longer the same. There now is a clear before and after. Now, everything makes me tired.

But I refuse to give in. I have started to travel again in an effort to fulfill my commitments. I try not to cancel engagements, conferences, except if they entail long trips. I listen to Marion: no more impulsive promises.

However, I have had to reduce my presence at the university: The weekly courses were too exhausting, as were the frequent New York–Boston trips. And the preparation of my three public lectures in the fall takes more of my time. It now takes me hours of research to gather the material for my lectures at the 92nd Street Y in Manhattan, lectures such as "Why I Love Isaac" or "Thoughts on Good and Evil in the Jewish Tradition." There are still so many subjects to tackle; I tell myself that, somehow, I have just begun.

I continue to revel in the search for the secret truths hidden in ancient and immortal texts. And in their interpretations, drawn from the imaginary more than from memory.

When this book was published in France, I was surprised: It appeared to be doing better than I was. It even found a spot on the bestseller list. Why this sudden success? I don't even try to understand. Like authors, books have their own destiny.

The physical pains are less intense but have not disappeared entirely. If I forget them for a while, they quickly remind me of their presence.

My two grandchildren continue to be a constant source of strength and joy. As I watch them grow, I desperately want to keep the promise to my son, Elisha: to be present at Elijah's bar mitzvah and perhaps even at Shira's bat mitzvah. I have already been the beneficiary of so many miracles, which I know I owe to my ancestors. All I have achieved has been and continues to be dedicated to their murdered dreams—and hopes.

I am infinitely grateful to them.

My life? I go on breathing from minute to minute, from prayer to prayer.

ACKNOWLEDGMENTS

With deepest gratitude I thank my doctors:

    Dr. Nirav Patel

    Dr. Howard Cohen

    Dr. Charles Friedlander

    Dr. David Seinfeld

    Dr. Stephen D. Nimer

Their devoted care pulled me from the edge.

                               E.W.

A NOTE ABOUT THE AUTHOR

Elie Wiesel was fifteen years old when he was deported to Auschwitz. He became a journalist and writer in Paris after the war, and since then has written more than fifty books, fiction and nonfiction, including his masterwork, *Night,* a major best seller when it was republished recently in a new translation. He has been awarded the United States Congressional Gold Medal, the Presidential Medal of Freedom, the rank of Grand Cross in the French Legion of Honor, an honorary knighthood of the British Empire and, in 1986, the Nobel Peace Prize. Since 1976, he has been the Andrew W. Mellon Professor in the Humanities at Boston University.

A NOTE ON THE TYPE

The text of this book was set in Sabon, a type-
face designed by Jan Tschichold (1902–1974),
the well-known German typographer. Based
loosely on the original designs by Claude Gara-
mond (c. 1480–1561), Sabon is unique in that
it was explicitly designed for hot-metal com-
position on both the Monotype and Linotype
machines as well as for filmsetting. Designed
in 1966 in Frankfurt, Sabon was named for
the famous Lyons punch cutter Jacques Sabon,
who is thought to have brought some of Gara-
mond's matrices to Frankfurt.

Composed by North Market Street Graphics
Lancaster, Pennsylvania

Printed and bound by Berryville Graphics
Berryville, Virginia

Designed by Maggie Hinders